UPDOG

DEADLY DISEASES

EBOLA

A Rare Killer

Jackie Golusky

Lerner Publications ◆ Minneapolis

Lerner Publications Company
An imprint of Lerner Publishing Group, Inc.
241 First Avenue North
Minneapolis, MN 55401 USA

For reading levels and more information, look up this title at www.lernerbooks.com.

Main body text set in ITC Franklin Gothic Std.
Typeface provided by Adobe Systems.

Designer: Mary Ross

Library of Congress Cataloging-in-Publication Data

Names: Golusky, Jackie, 1996– author.
Title: Ebola : a rare killer / Jackie Golusky.
Description: Minneapolis: Lerner Publications, [2022] | Series: Deadly diseases (Updog books) | Includes bibliographical references and index. | Audience: Ages 8–11 | Audience: Grades 2–3 | Summary: "Learn how scientists and doctors identify and treat Ebola fever, an often deadly disease caused by the Ebola virus"— Provided by publisher.
Identifiers: LCCN 2020049999 (print) | LCCN 2020050000 (ebook) | ISBN 9781728428338 (library binding) | ISBN 9781728431246 (paperback) | ISBN 9781728430607 (ebook)
Subjects: LCSH: Ebola virus disease—Juvenile literature. | Epidemics—Juvenile literature.
Classification: LCC RC140.5 .G66 2022 (print) | LCC RC140.5 (ebook) | DDC 614.5/88—dc23

LC record available at https://lccn.loc.gov/2020049999
LC ebook record available at https://lccn.loc.gov/2020050000

Manufactured in the United States of America
1-49370-49474-2/25/2021

Table of Contents

A Dangerous Disease 4

Outbreak 11

Up Close 12

Stopping the Spread 16

Doctor You! 21

Glossary 22

Check It Out! 23

Index 24

A Dangerous Disease

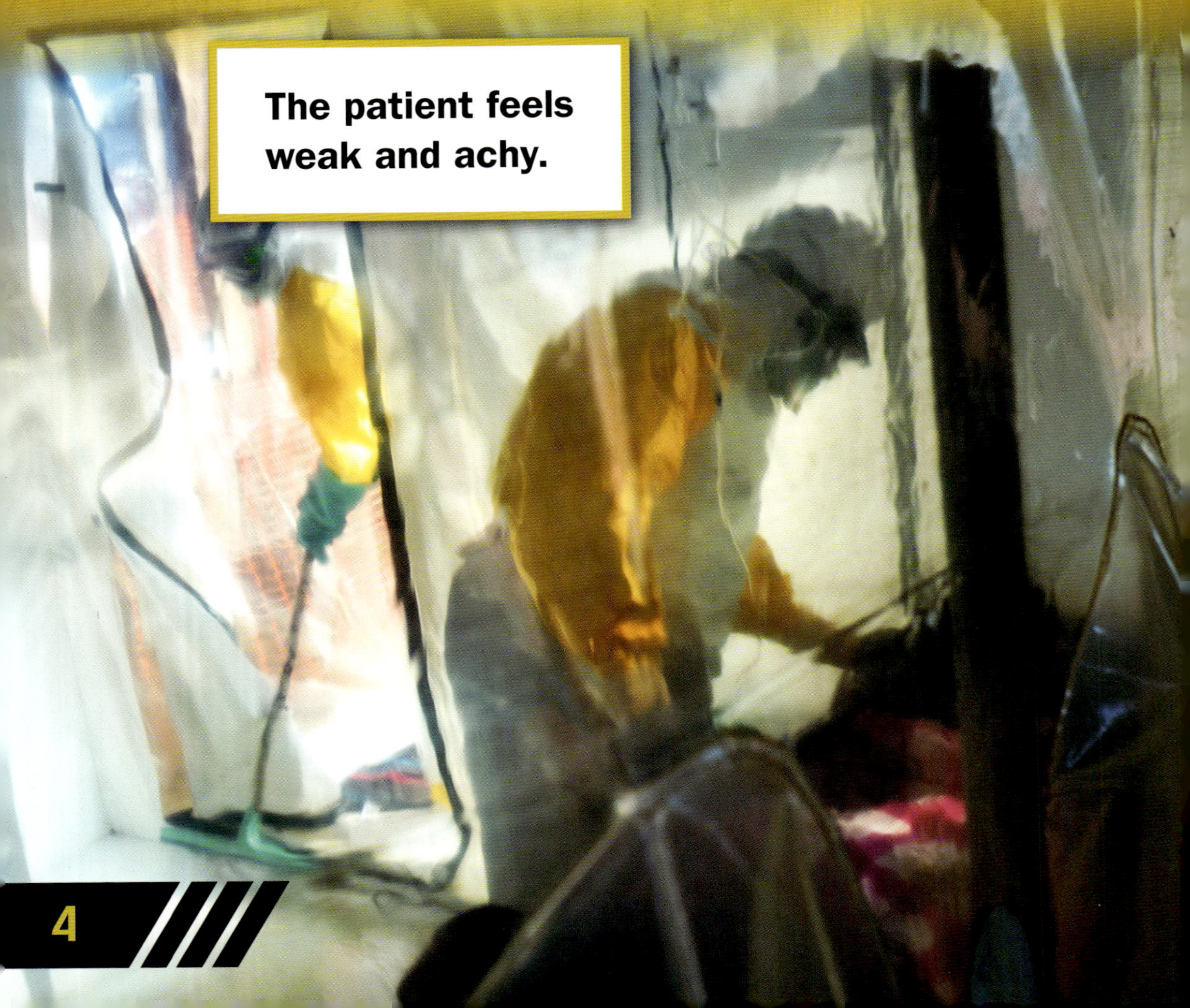

The patient feels weak and achy.

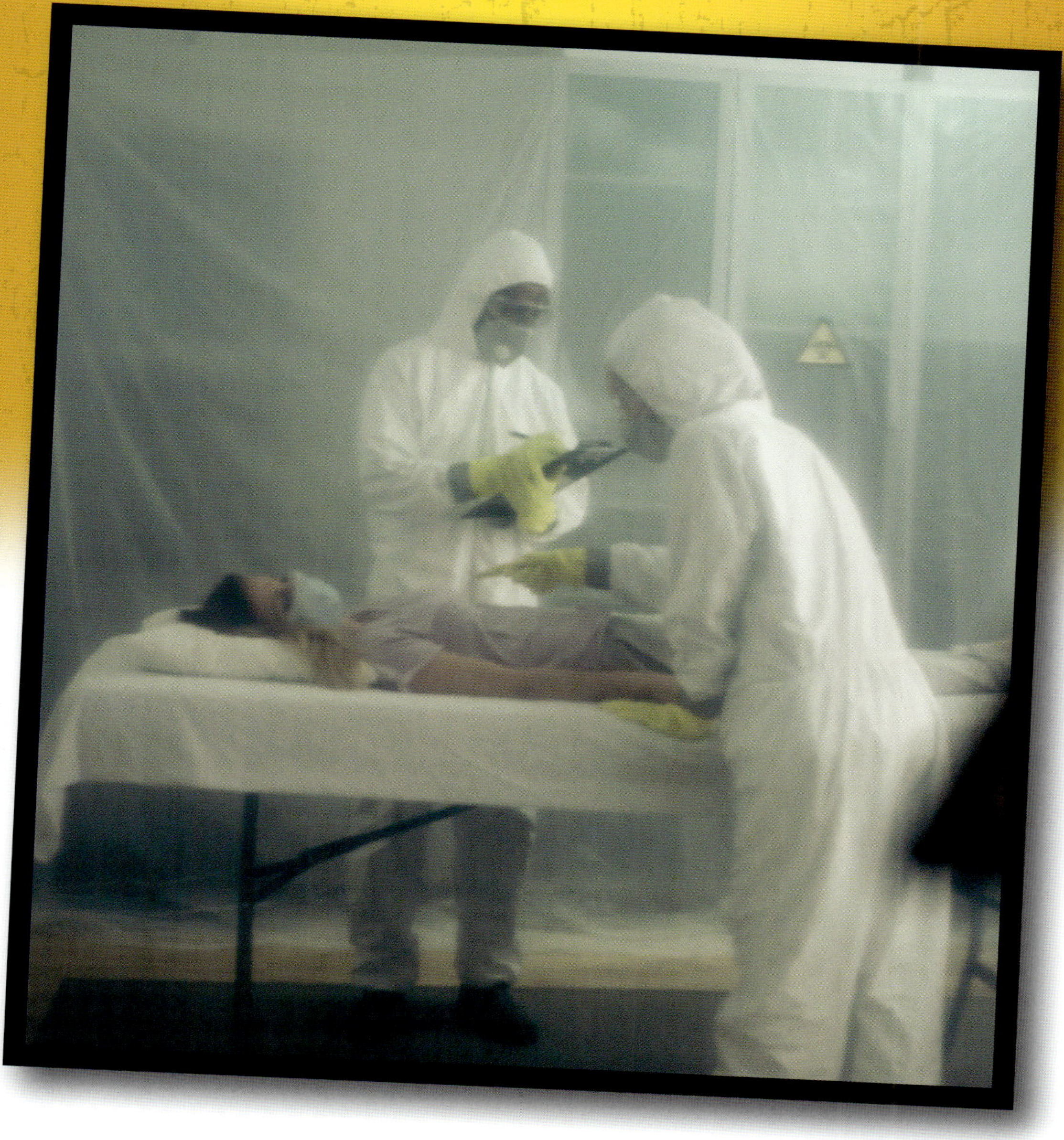

She has a fever and red eyes.

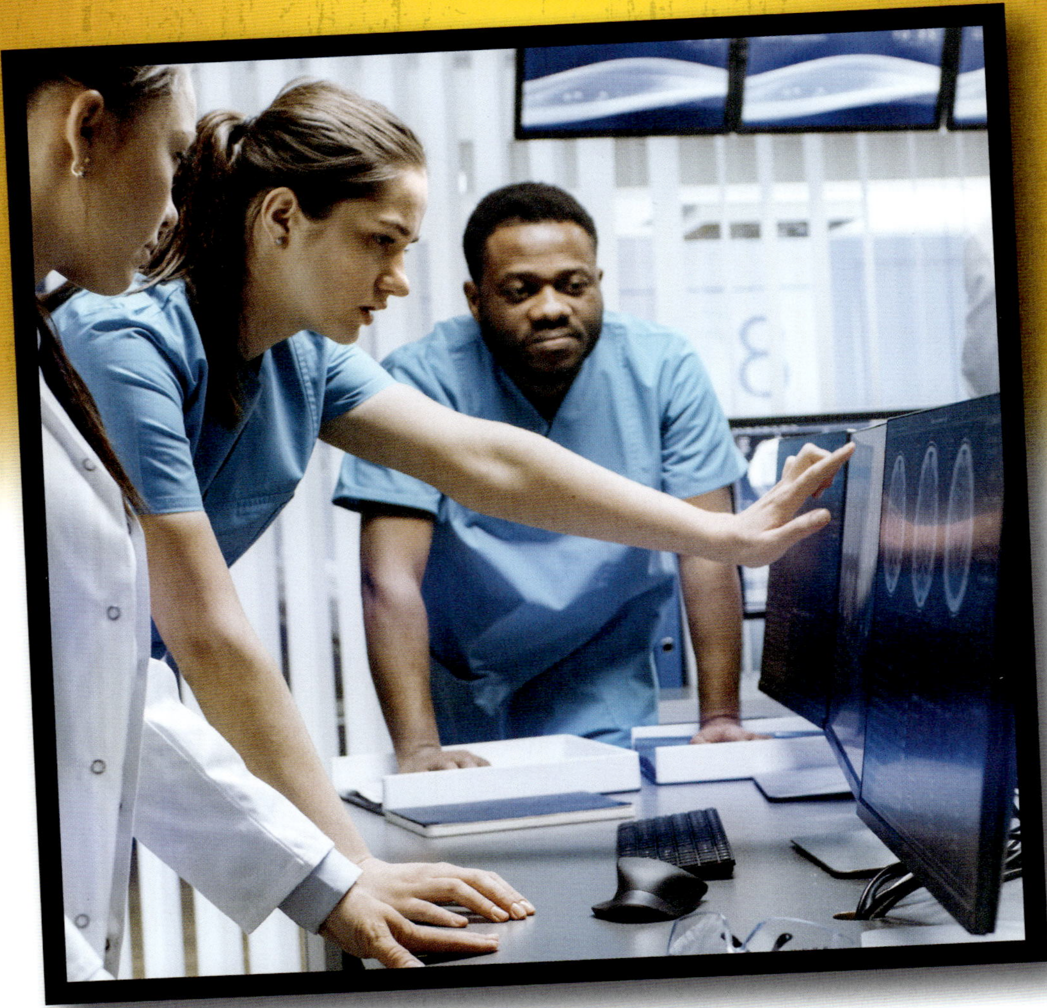

Doctors say she has Ebola.

A virus causes the disease.

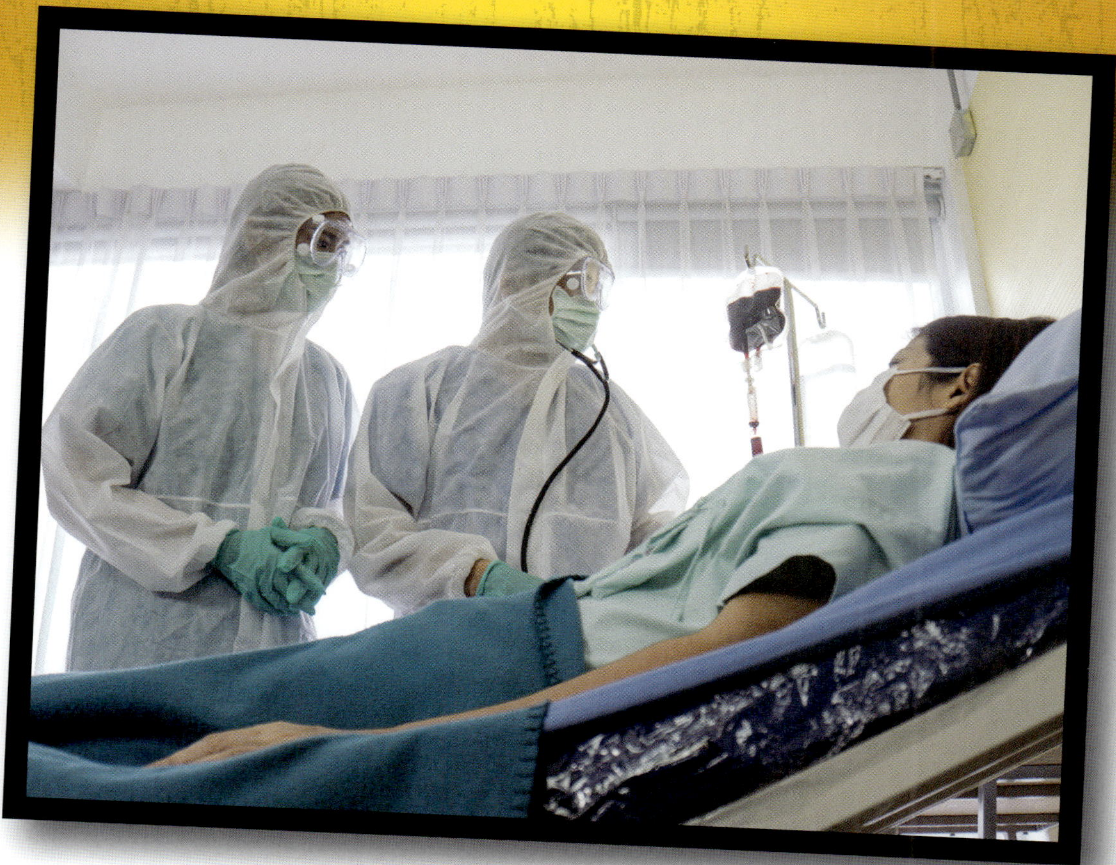

virus: a tiny thing that causes disease

The virus enters through the eyes, nose, or mouth.

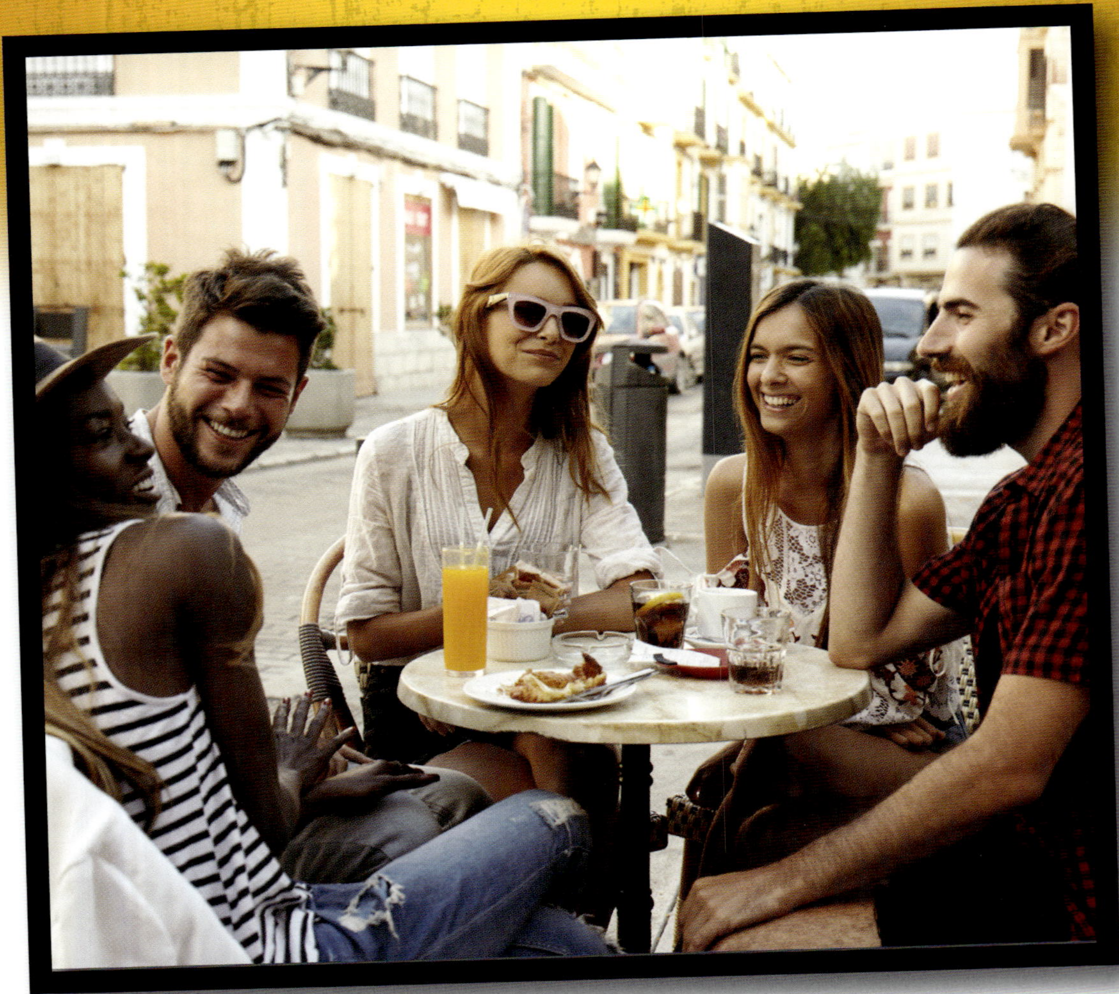

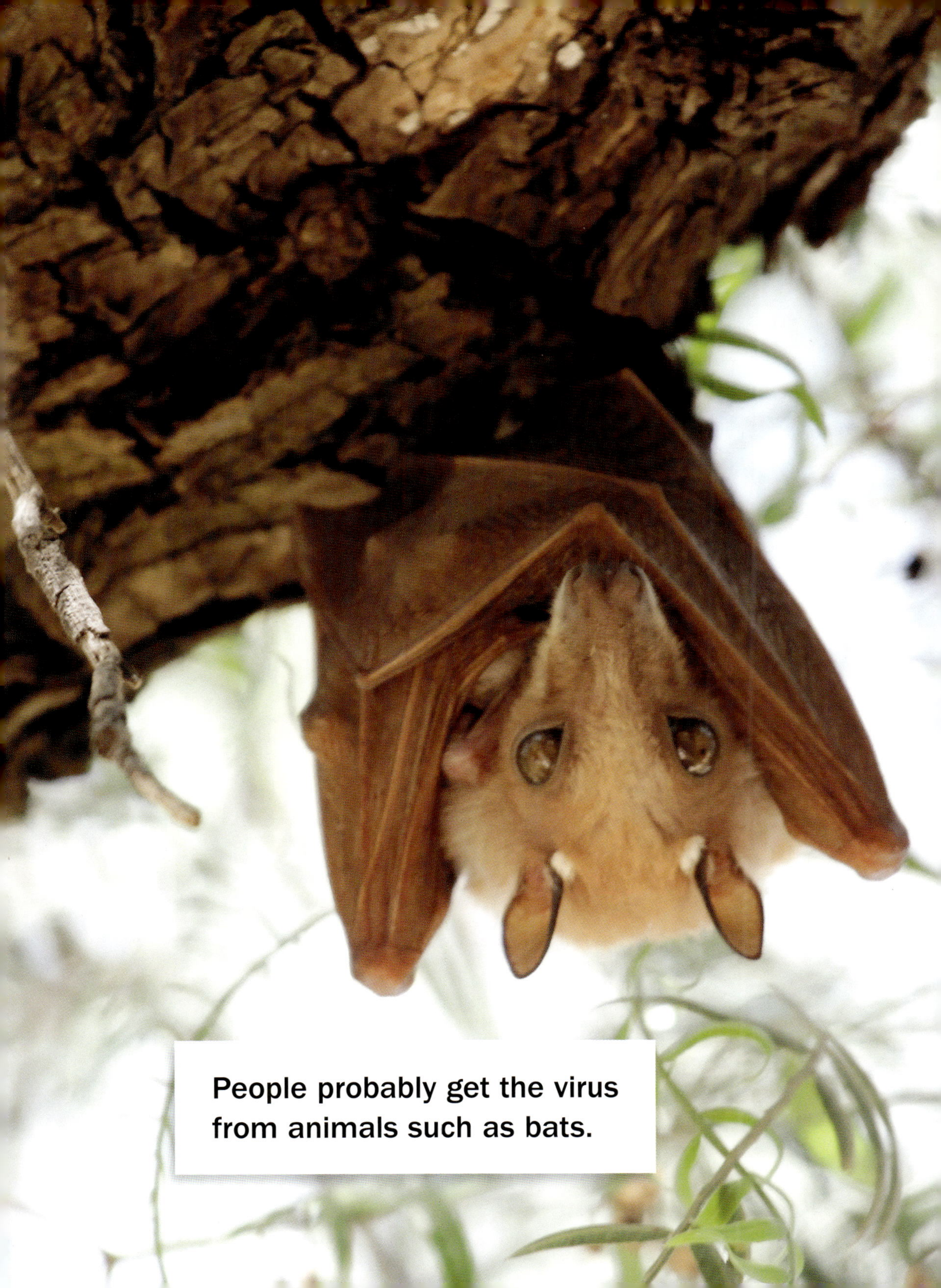

People probably get the virus from animals such as bats.

Then it spreads from person to person.

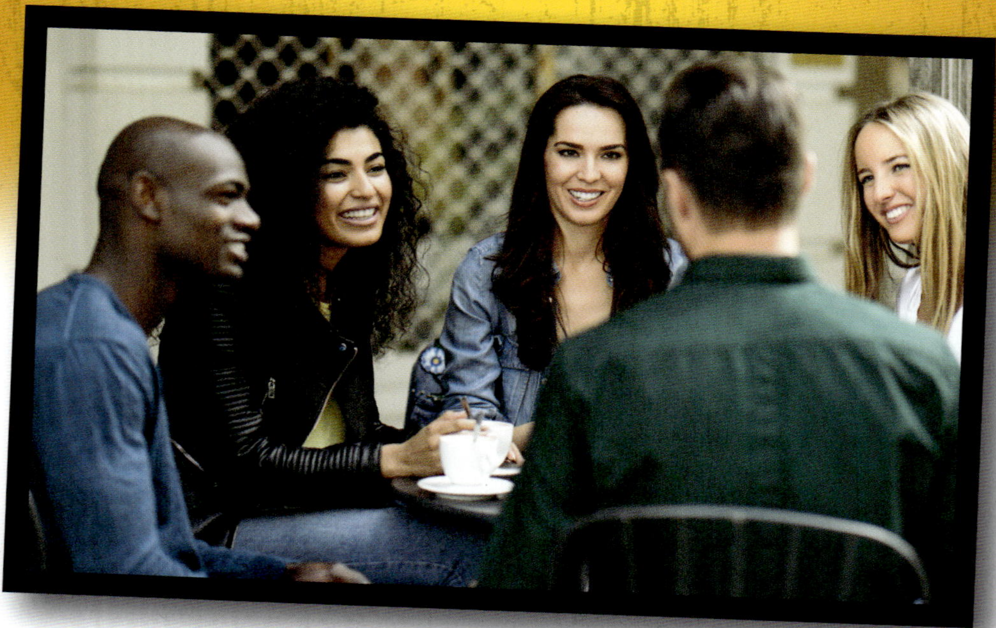

UP NEXT!

Rising Cases.

Outbreak

In 2014–2016, an Ebola outbreak happened.

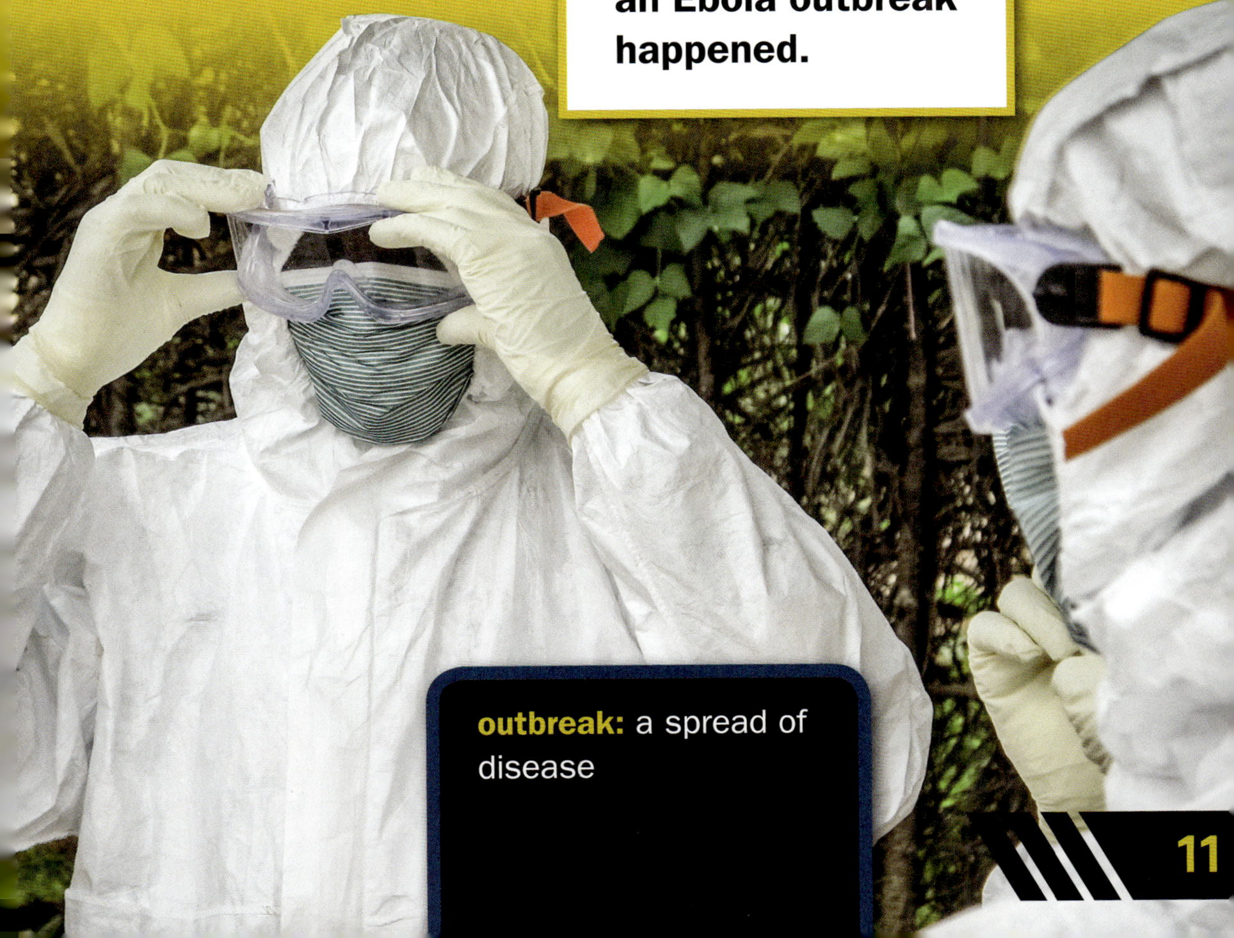

outbreak: a spread of disease

UP CLOSE

The image on the right shows the Ebola virus.

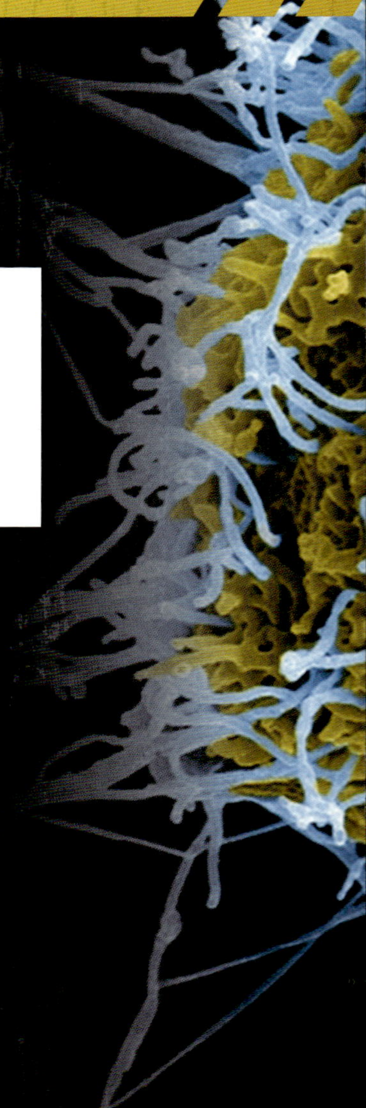

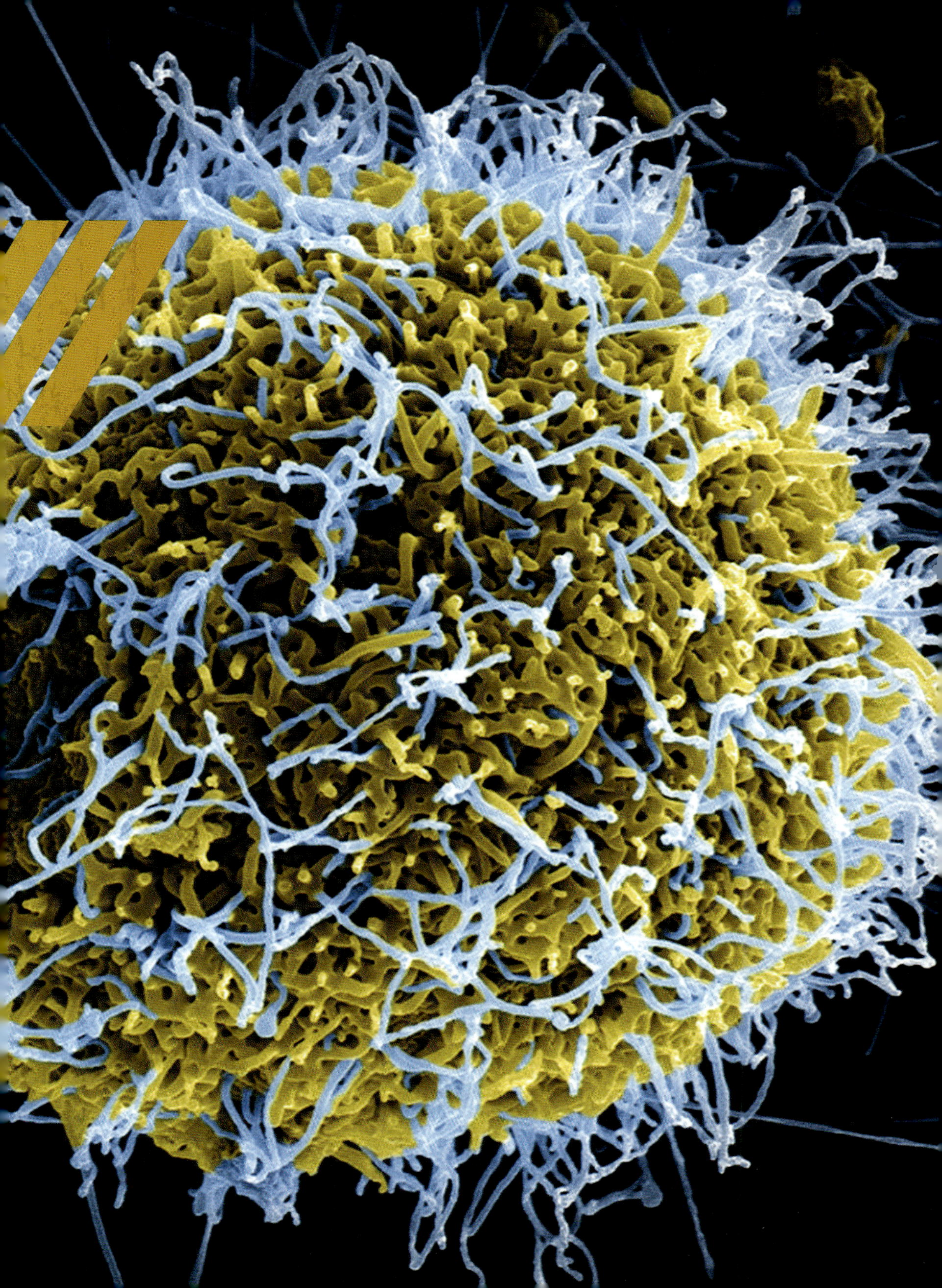

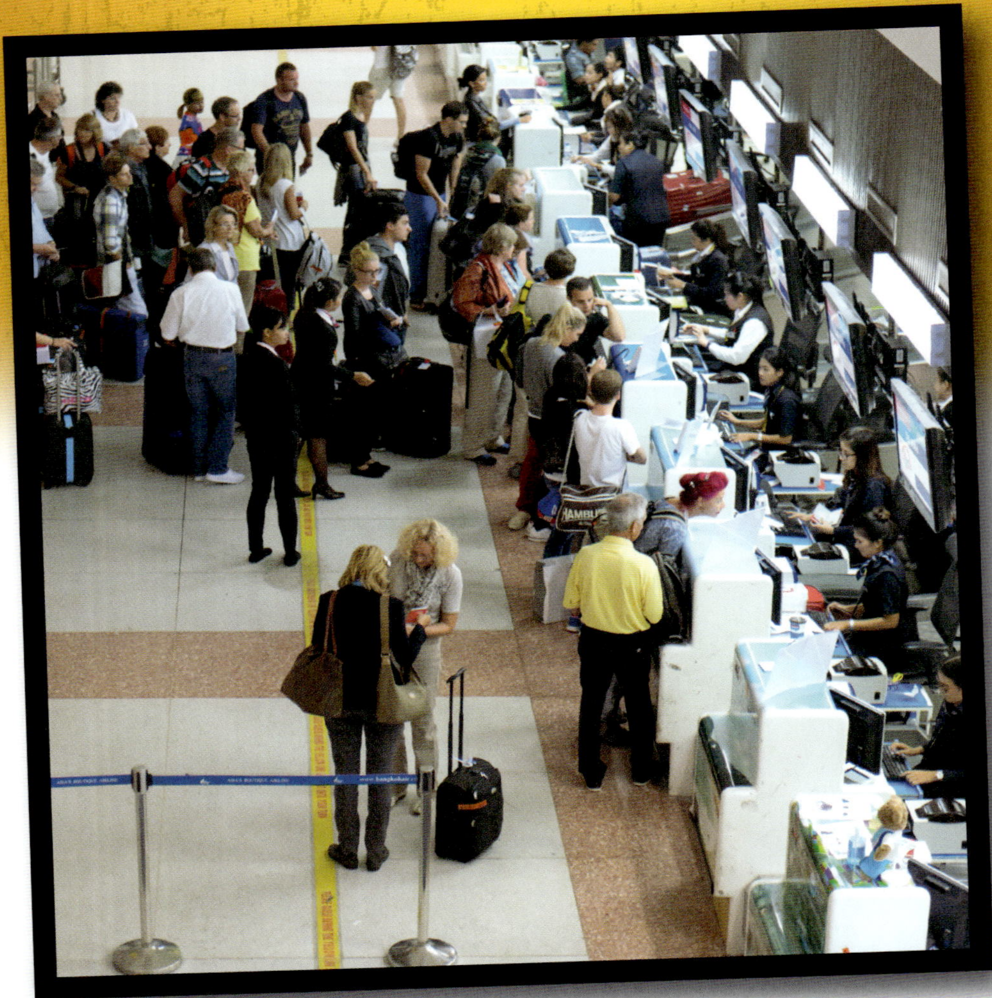

Ebola spread around the world.

Many people died from the disease.

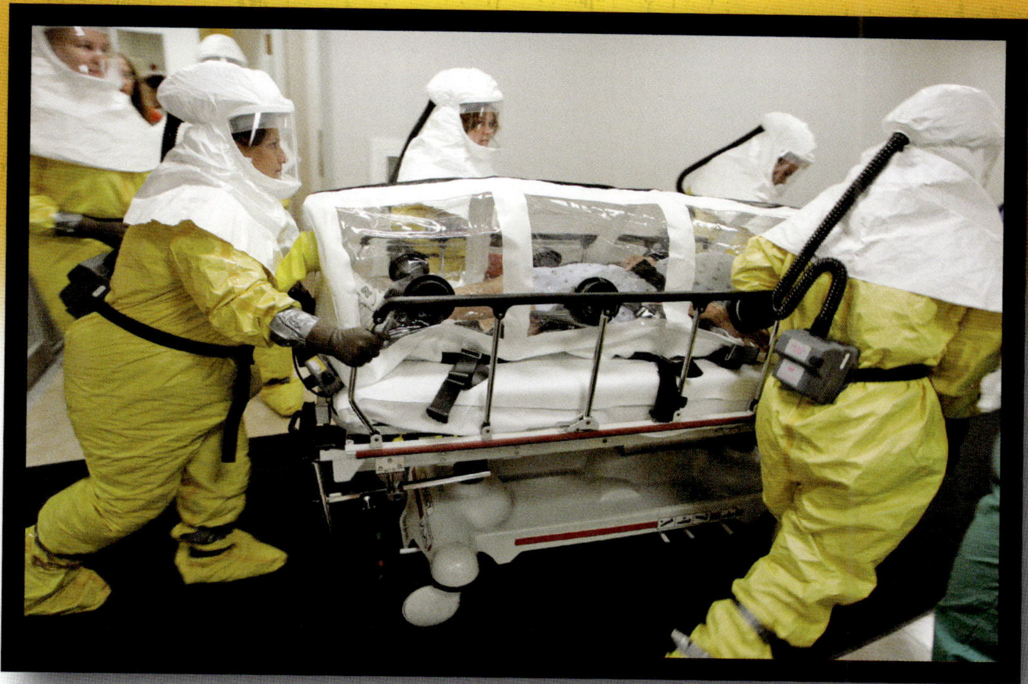

UP NEXT!

Testing and Treatment.

Stopping the Spread

Scientists are working on an Ebola vaccine.

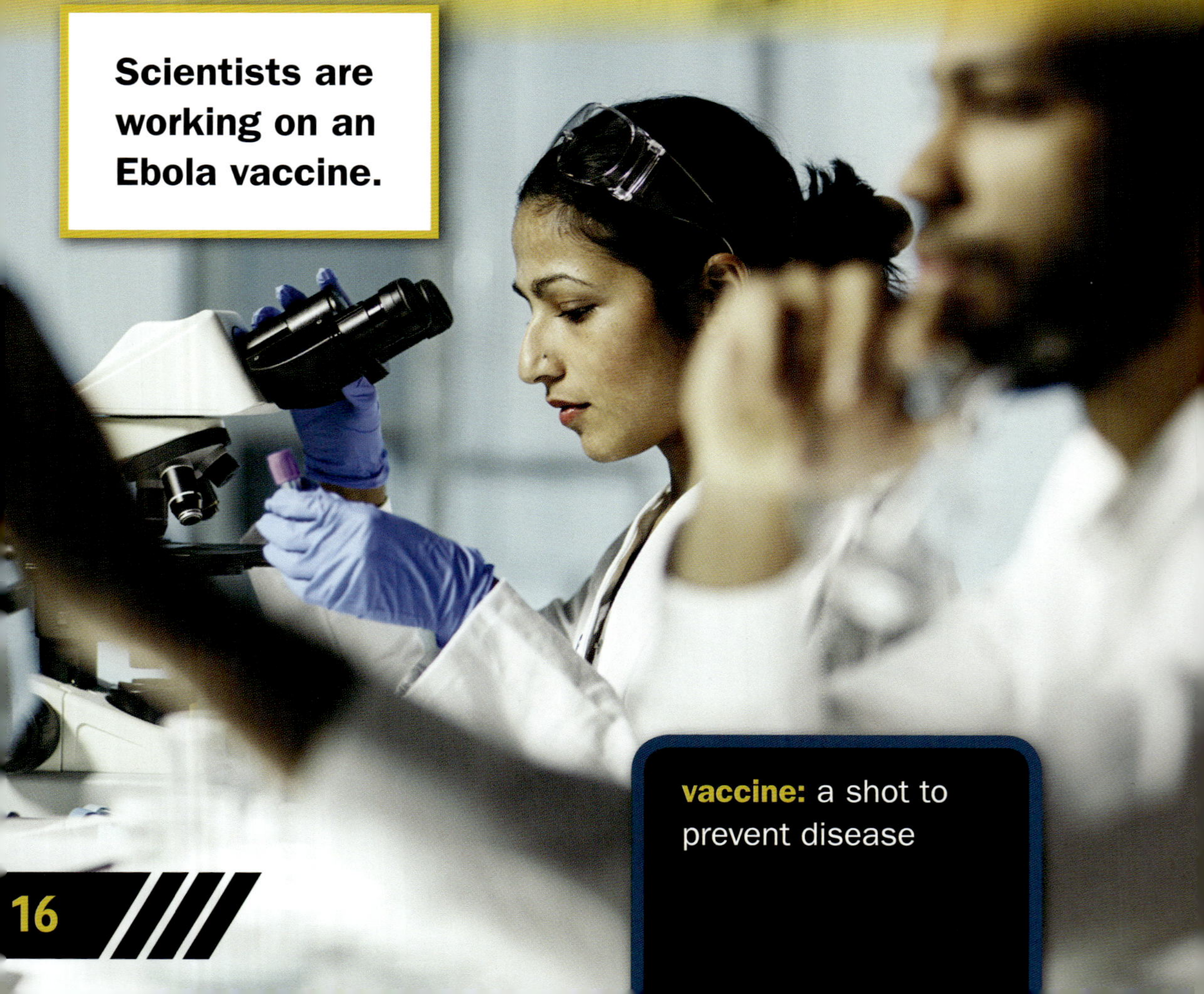

vaccine: a shot to prevent disease

It would stop people from getting the disease.

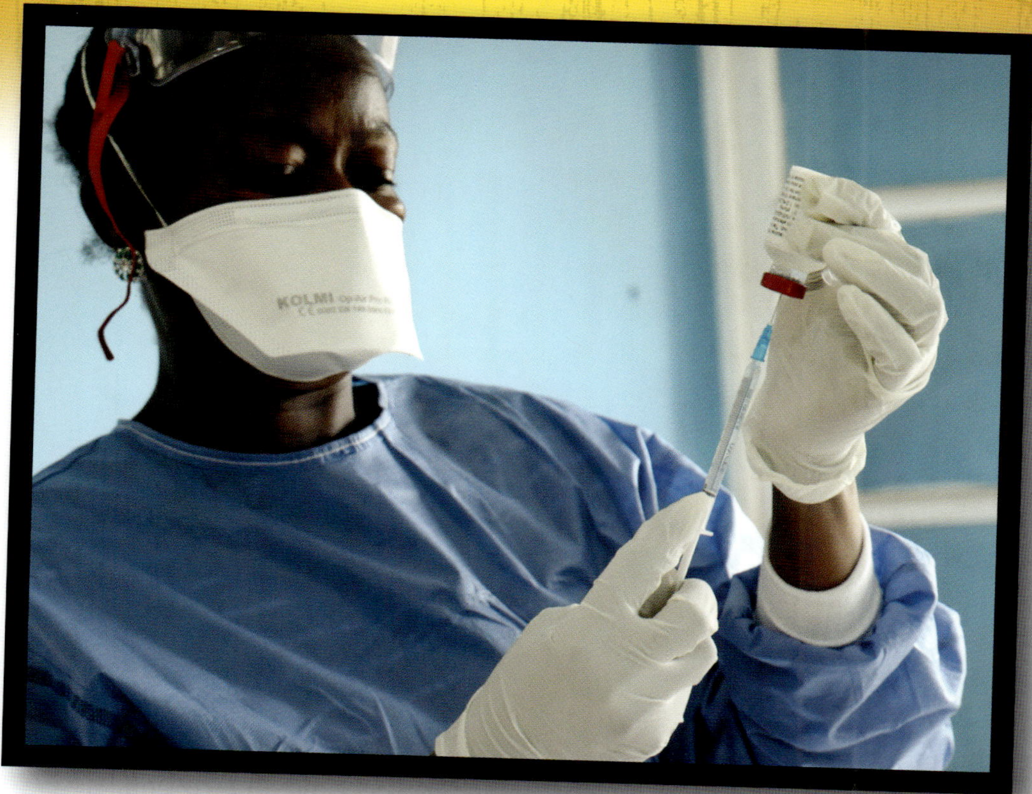

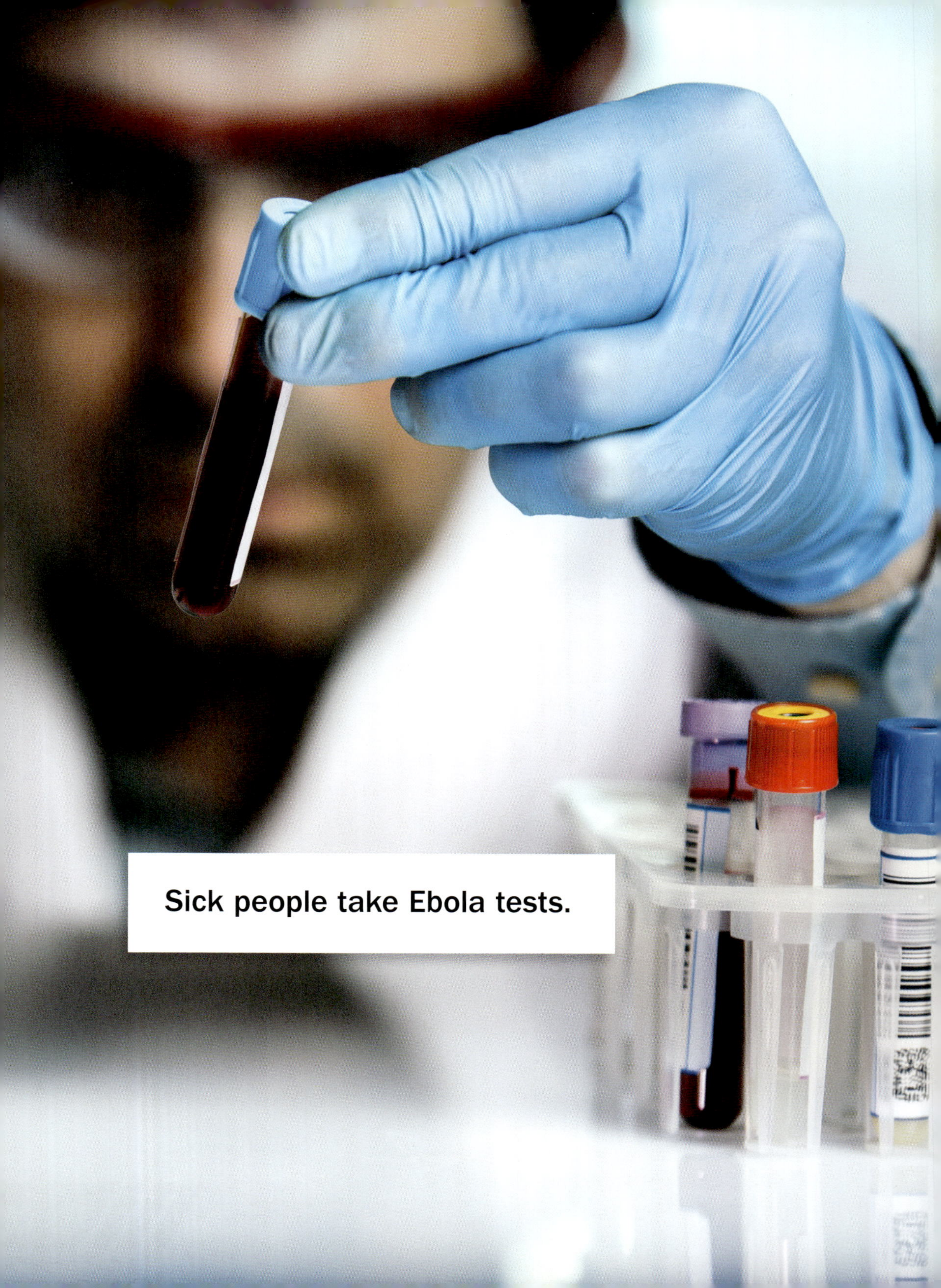

Sick people take Ebola tests.

Doctors and nurses help people who have the disease.

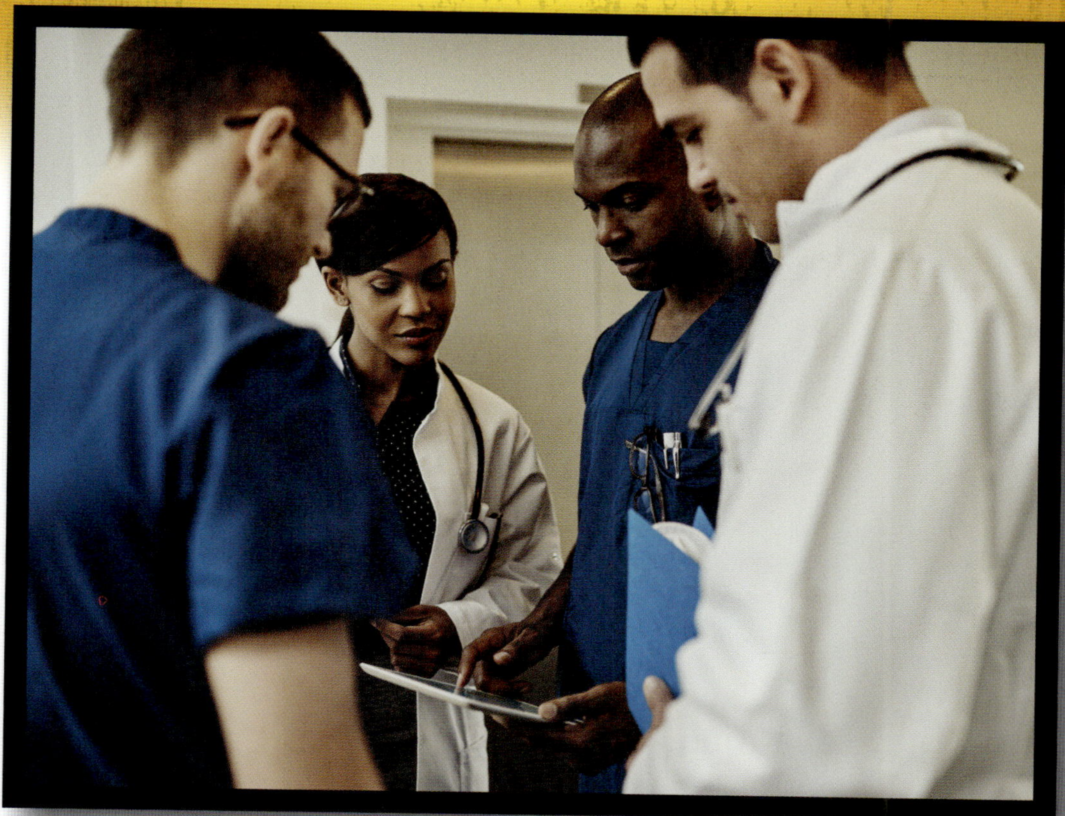

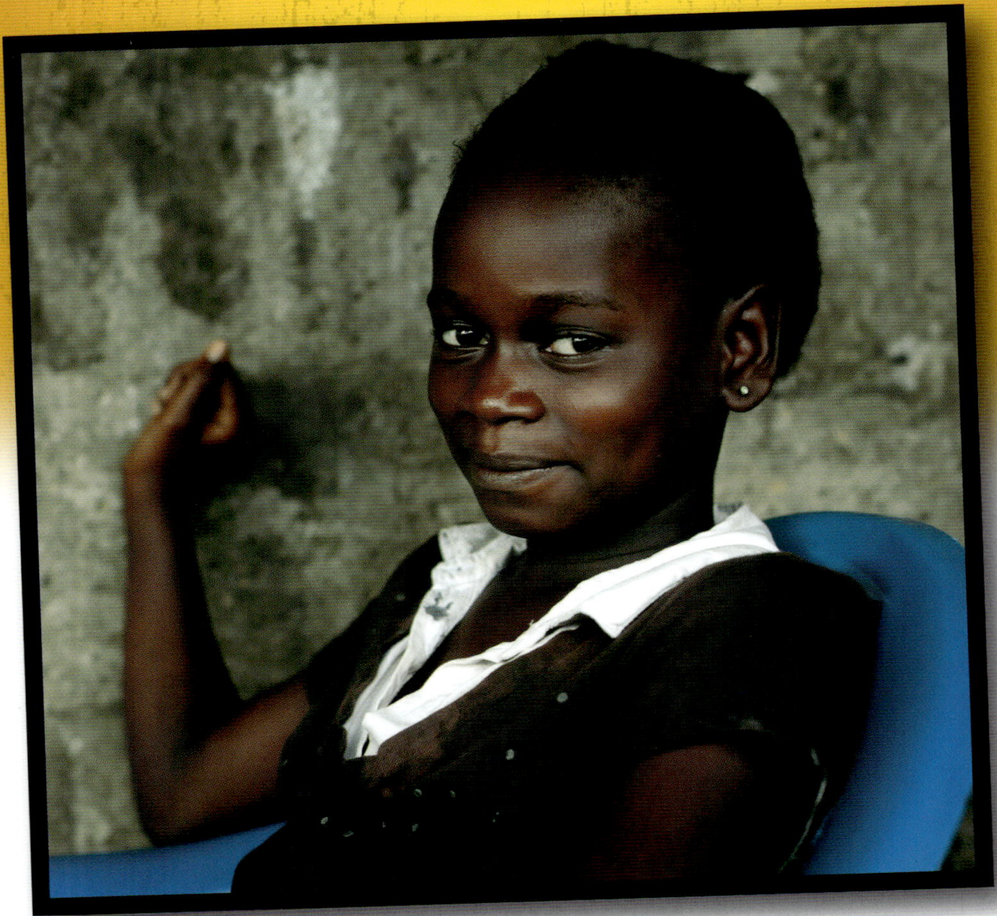

They save many lives.

DOCTOR YOU!

Which patient has Ebola?

Patient A

red eyes
aches
fever

Patient B

aches
cough
fever

Answer: Patient A

Glossary

outbreak: a spread of disease

vaccine: a shot to prevent disease

virus: a tiny thing that causes disease

Check It Out!

Abdo, Kenny. *Ebola Outbreak*. Minneapolis: Abdo, 2021.

Britannica Kids: Ebola
https://kids.britannica.com/kids/article/Ebola/610103

Hudak, Heather C. *Ebola*. New York: AV2, 2020.

Kaiser, Brianna. *Smallpox: A Vaccine Success*. Minneapolis: Lerner Publications, 2022.

KidsHealth: What Are Germs?
https://kidshealth.org/en/kids/germs.html

Science News for Students: What Is Ebola?
https://www.sciencenewsforstudents.org/article/explainer-what-ebola

Index

doctors, 6, 19

fever, 5

outbreak, 11

red eyes, 5

spread, 10–11, 14

vaccine, 16

virus, 7–9, 12

Photo Acknowledgments

Image credits: AP Photo/Jerome Delay, p. 4; David Pereiras/Alamy Stock Photo, p. 5; Gorodenkoff/Shutterstock.com, p. 6; sandyman/Shutterstock.com, p. 7; Monkey Business Images/Shutterstock.com, p. 8; weisschr/iStock/Getty Images, p. 9; javi_indy/Shutterstock.com, p. 10; AP Photo/Michael Duff, p. 11; National Institutes of Health, p9. 12-13; AP Photo/Stephen Wandera, p. 14; Iryna Rasko/Shutterstock.com, p. 15; poba/E+/Getty Images, p. 16; AP Photo/Sam Mednick, p. 17; angellodeco/Shutterstock.com, p. 18; Flamingo Images/Shutterstock.com, p. 19; AP Photo/Jerome Delay, p. 20.

Cover: Festa/Shutterstock.com.